The Truth About Brain Food

How to Separate Fact from Fiction and Choose the Best Diet for Your Mind

By

Rawley D. Crepeau

DISCLAIMER

Copyright © by Rawley D. Crepeau 2024. All rights reserved. Before this document is duplicated or reproduced in any manner, the publisher's consent must be gained. Therefore, the contents within can neither be stored electronically, transferred, nor kept in a database. Neither in Part nor full can the document be copied, scanned, faxed, or retained without approval from the publisher or creator.

Contents

Introduction

How Your Brain Is Shaped by Food
Your brain is impacted by the food you consume in addition to your body. Your mood, memory, cognitive function, and even your chance of developing neurodegenerative disorders can all be impacted by the food you eat. But how can one determine what to eat for maximum brain health when there is so much contradicting and confusing information available?
This book will teach you the real deal about brain food, the science behind brain metabolism, and the benefits of individualized eating. You will discover the truths behind the hype around antioxidants, plant-based diets, superfoods, and supplements. You will also gain insight into the relationship between brain health and insulin

resistance, ketones, and essential fatty acids. Additionally, you will discover how to assess the state of your brain, select the healthiest diet for your brain, and optimize your diet for your brain. This book is for everyone who wishes to use food's power to protect, revitalize, and feed their brain. You can enhance your brain health with food, regardless of your age, health, or preference for meat- or plant-based diets. Our guidance is grounded in science and practical experience. You will have a thorough understanding of how food affects your brain and how to modify your diet for optimal brain function by the end of this book.

Part I: The Truth About Brain Food

Brain food: what is it? Is there a certain kind of diet that improves cognition, memory, and brain power? Is it a supplement that can stop or slow Alzheimer's and cognitive decline? Is there a diet that can improve your creativity, happiness, and intelligence? None of the above is the response.

Brain food doesn't exist. No single meal, dietary supplement, or way of eating can ensure ideal brain function and health. In actuality, some of the most well-known and overhyped brain meals are unproven, based on exaggerated or incorrect claims, or even detrimental to your brain, according to scientific research.

In this chapter, we will dispel some of the most widespread misconceptions around brain food, including:

The falsehood about supplements and superfoods: why taking vitamins, antioxidants, or nootropics won't keep your brain healthy as you age or get sick, and why eating blueberries, walnuts, or fish oil won't make you a genius.

The misconception about plant-based diets Why giving up meat, dairy, or eggs won't stop or reverse Alzheimer's disease; and why adopting a vegan, vegetarian, or gluten-free diet won't make you smarter, happier, or more creative.

The myth of antioxidants: why taking antioxidant supplements or pills may potentially be detrimental to your brain, and why increasing your intake of antioxidants won't shield your brain from oxidative stress or free radicals.

We'll also discuss the truth about brain food using the most recent data and scientific studies. We will demonstrate how food influences your brain's metabolism—the process by which your brain absorbs and utilizes the energy and nutrients from the food you eat—rather than offering mystical or miraculous effects.

We'll demonstrate how various food kinds impact your brain's metabolism in many ways, including:

How insulin resistance, inflammation, and oxidative stress caused by carbs, particularly refined sugars and starches, can affect brain metabolism and result in neurodegeneration, mood disorders, and cognitive decline.

how fats, particularly omega-3 fatty acids, can boost your brain's metabolism by offering a different and more effective energy source, and how this can benefit your mood, cognitive abilities, and neuroprotection.

Proteins, particularly important amino acids, can help your brain's metabolism by acting as the building blocks for hormones, enzymes, and neurotransmitters; this can control your mood, neuroplasticity, and cognitive function.

Additionally, we will demonstrate how to apply the science of brain metabolism to your nutrition by offering you customized, actionable guidance on selecting the optimal diet for your brain, taking into account your unique needs, preferences, and objectives.

We'll teach you how to optimize your food for mental health by adhering to a few straightforward guidelines, like:

Consuming a diet rich in fruits, vegetables, legumes, whole grains, and dairy products in moderation, along with reasonable amounts of fish, poultry, eggs, dairy products, nuts, and seeds.

Steer clear of or consume fewer processed and junk foods, which are lacking in fiber, vitamins, minerals, and phytochemicals and rich in sugar, salt, fat, additives, and preservatives.

consuming adequate amounts of water and other healthful liquids, including juice, tea, or coffee, while limiting or abstaining from soda, alcohol, and energy drinks.

Eating by your body's signals of hunger and fullness; refraining from bingeing, fasting, overeating, or skipping meals or snacks.

eating with enjoyment and mindfulness, avoiding distractions, stress, or guilt.

You will nourish, safeguard, and invigorate your body as well as your general health and well-being by adhering to these guidelines.

In conclusion, the truth regarding brain food is that it doesn't exist. There is only food, and food influences your brain by altering its metabolism rather than working magic or performing miracles. You may enhance both the health and function of your brain and your enjoyment of food by learning how food influences brain metabolism and designing and adjusting your diet accordingly.

Chapter 1: The Myth of Superfoods and Supplements

Supplements and superfoods are frequently promoted as the best options for overall health and well-being. They offer a host of advantages, including increased immunity, disease prevention, performance enhancement, and longevity promotion. But are these assertions supported by data from science, or are they merely marketing speak?

Although there isn't a formal meaning for the phrase "superfood," it usually refers to foods high in antioxidants, nutrients, or other substances thought to have health benefits. Several foods are frequently referred to as superfoods, including salmon, quinoa, kale, blueberries, and turmeric. Nevertheless, there isn't enough evidence to say that any of these foods are better for you nutritionally than other foods or that they can prevent or treat any particular ailment. As a matter of fact, there can be disadvantages to some superfoods, such as excessive calorie, sugar, or oxalate content, which can lead to kidney stones.

Comparably, the word "supplement" refers to a broad category of goods, including probiotics, vitamins, minerals, herbs, amino acids, and enzymes. Certain populations require specific supplements, such as vegans, expectant mothers, and people with illnesses that interfere with the body's ability to absorb nutrients. However, supplements are not necessary and may even be hazardous for the majority of healthy adults who consume a balanced diet. Overdosing on some supplements might have negative consequences like nausea, diarrhea, liver damage, or drug interactions.

Furthermore, the Food and Drug Administration (FDA) does not regulate supplements, so there is no assurance of their efficacy, safety, or quality. Ultimately, superfoods and supplements cannot take the place of a healthy lifestyle; they are not miracle cures. The body cannot be supplied with all the nutrients and advantages it requires by a single diet or medication. Eating a range of meals from various food categories, limiting processed and junk food, drinking lots of water, exercising frequently, getting enough sleep, and managing stress are the greatest ways to reach maximum health. Developing these behaviors is more efficient and long-lasting than depending solely on supplements and superfoods that might not be as beneficial as advertised.

Foods high in antioxidants, minerals, and other health-promoting substances that may help prevent or treat a variety of ailments are a few examples of superfoods. Several popular superfoods consist of:

Rich in fiber, vitamins, minerals, and phytochemicals, dark leafy vegetables like kale, spinach, and collard greens may lower the chance of developing chronic conditions like cancer, diabetes, and heart disease.

Berries rich in antioxidants and fiber, such as blueberries, raspberries, and cranberries, may offer protection against oxidative stress, inflammation, and digestive issues.

Omega-3 fatty acids and protein-rich fish, such as sardines, tuna, and salmon, may help the immune system, heart health, and brain function.

Nuts rich in protein, good fats, and minerals that may reduce blood pressure, inflammation, and cholesterol include walnuts, pecans, and almonds.

High in monounsaturated fat, vitamin E, and polyphenols, olive oil may help blood vessels work better, reduce cholesterol, and fend off oxidative damage.

Whole grains are rich in fiber, vitamins, minerals, and phytochemicals that may help control blood sugar, decrease cholesterol, and prevent diabetes. Examples of these grains are brown rice, quinoa, and oats.

Superfoods come in a wide variety of forms, so keep in mind that no one food can give you all the health advantages you require. Eating a range of whole foods from various food groups and speaking with a certified specialist before taking any supplements are the best ways to make the most out of your diet.

Some benefits of eating superfoods are: They provide a high amount of nutrients and antioxidants that may help prevent or treat various diseases, such as heart disease, cancer, diabetes, and inflammation.

They support the health and function of different organs and systems in the body, such as the heart, brain, immune system, digestive system, and skin.

They may enhance your mood, energy, and cognitive performance by influencing your hormones, blood sugar, and neurotransmitters.

They may help you maintain a healthy weight by providing fiber, protein, and healthy fats that can keep you full and satisfied.

However, it is important to remember that superfoods are not a substitute for a balanced and varied diet. They are best consumed as part of a healthy lifestyle that includes other whole foods, physical activity, and stress management.

Chapter 2: The Myth of Plant-Based Diets

Diets based mostly on plants are growing in popularity as more individuals look to enhance their health, save the environment, and lessen the suffering of animals. But there are also a lot of false beliefs and misconceptions regarding plant-based diets that could discourage or perplex some individuals who would like to follow this way of life. In this post, we'll dispel some of the most widespread misconceptions regarding plant-based diets and offer some data-backed advice.

Myth 1: Diets based solely on plants are inadequate in calcium, iron, protein, and other nutrients.

The idea that plant-based diets are insufficient in key nutrients—particularly protein, iron, calcium, and vitamin B12—is one of the most pervasive misunderstandings about them. This is untrue, though, if the diet is balanced and well-planned. In addition to additional health-promoting vitamins, minerals, antioxidants, and phytochemicals, plant-based diets can equal or surpass recommended intakes of these nutrients. Amino acids, the building blocks of muscles, tissues, hormones, enzymes, and antibodies, make up protein, a macronutrient. Nine of the twenty amino acids are considered essential, indicating that the body cannot produce them on its own and must get them from diet. Because animal products like meat, eggs, and dairy contain all nine essential amino acids in sufficient amounts, they are regarded as complete proteins. But as long as they are ingested in a variety of forms and sufficient quantities, plant-based foods can likewise offer sufficient amounts and quality of protein.

A few plant-based foods that contain all nine essential amino acids are called complete proteins, and these include soy, quinoa, buckwheat, hemp seeds, and chia seeds. Other plant foods include grains, beans, lentils, nuts, seeds, vegetables, and legumes; these foods are incomplete proteins since they either don't contain any necessary amino acids at all or have very little of them. That does not, however, imply that they are less valuable or insignificant. You can get all the required amino acids at a meal or throughout the day by mixing diverse plant foods, like peanut butter and toast, hummus and pita bread, or beans and rice.

0.8 grams of protein per kilogram of body weight per day is the recommended dietary allowance (RDA) for adults, or roughly 56 grams for men and 46 grams for women. This is not an ideal intake but rather a minimal requirement, and it can change based on goals, age, activity level, and health. According to some experts, older folks, athletes, and those looking to grow muscle or lose weight may benefit from consuming up to 1.2 grams of protein per kilogram of body weight every day.

Plant-based diets can readily achieve both the greater intake recommended by some experts and the RDA for protein. The amount of protein in a cup of cooked lentils is 18, the amount in a cup of cooked quinoa is 8, the amount in a quarter cup of almonds is 8, and the amount in a cup of soy milk is 7. Consuming a diverse range of plant-based foods throughout the day can readily provide an adequate amount of protein to support both health and performance.

The mineral iron is needed to make red blood cells, which are responsible for distributing oxygen throughout the body. Anemia, which is characterized by weakness, pale skin, weariness, and an increased risk of infection, can be brought on by an iron shortage. The recommended daily allowance (RDA) for iron is eight milligrams for men and eight milligrams for women. On the other hand, women who are nursing or pregnant require up to 27 mg of iron daily.

Heme and non-heme iron are the two forms found in food. Heme iron is more readily absorbed by the body and is exclusively present in animal items like meat, poultry, and fish. Both plant and animal items, including beans, lentils, tofu, spinach, kale, dried fruits, nuts, seeds, and fortified cereals, contain non-heme iron, although the body absorbs it more slowly. This does not imply, however, that diets based solely on plants lack iron. As long as plant-based diets are high in foods high in iron and supplemented with particular elements that promote iron absorption, they can supply sufficient levels of iron.

Vitamin C, which is found in large amounts in plant foods including citrus fruits, strawberries, kiwis, bell peppers, broccoli, and tomatoes, is one of the elements that can improve the absorption of iron. Consuming foods high in vitamin C in addition to foods high in iron can increase the absorption of non-heme iron by as much as six times. You can increase your intake of iron from these meals by, for instance, adding lemon juice to a spinach salad or sipping orange juice with a bowl of fortified cereal. Cooking with cast iron pots and pans, which can leach iron into the meal, particularly if the food is acidic like tomato sauce or vinegar, is another factor that might enhance the absorption of iron. You can add more iron to plant-based meals like stir-fries, stews, soups, and curries by using cast iron cookware.

However, other elements, including calcium, polyphenols, and phytates, can also reduce the absorption of iron. Whole grains, beans, nuts, and seeds contain substances called phytates that can bind to iron and prevent it from being absorbed. Antioxidants called polyphenols are present in tea, coffee, cocoa, and other spices. They can also obstruct the absorption of iron. Dairy products, fortified plant milks, and supplements include calcium, a mineral that may compete with iron for absorption. Increased iron intake from plant-based diets can be achieved by avoiding or reducing certain elements. Eating these foods at different times of the day than foods high in iron is one method to prevent or minimize these impacts. For instance, one can take calcium supplements at night rather than in the morning, or consume tea or coffee in between meals instead of with them.

Soaking, sprouting, or fermenting plant foods—such as grains, beans, nuts, and seeds—that include these components can also help prevent or minimize their effects by lowering phytate levels and increasing iron availability.

If plant-based diets are diversified and balanced, include foods high in iron and vitamin C, and use cast iron cookware, they can supply adequate levels of iron. Additionally, phytates, polyphenols, and calcium should be avoided or consumed in moderation.

Calcium is a necessary mineral for healthy bones, blood clotting, nerve transmission, and muscular contraction. Osteoporosis is a disorder marked by reduced bone density and an increased risk of fractures. It can be brought on by a calcium deficit. Persons should consume 1,000 mg of calcium daily, while older people should get 1,200 mg.

The most popular sources of calcium in the Western diet are dairy products, which include milk, cheese, and yogurt. These items are also frequently regarded as the best sources of calcium due to their high calcium content and excellent body absorption. Dairy products are not the only source of calcium, nor are they always the best option for all individuals. Some people may avoid dairy products for moral or environmental reasons, or they may be allergic, sensitive, or lactose intolerant. In these situations, plant-based diets—as long as they contain foods and supplements high in calcium—can supply sufficient levels of calcium.

Dark leafy greens, which may contain up to 250 mg of calcium per cup, such as bok choy, broccoli, collard greens, and kale, are among the plant foods high in calcium. Fortified plant milk, like soy, almond, oat, and rice milk, can offer up to 300 mg of calcium per cup, making them additional plant foods high in calcium. Tofu, tempeh, edamame, almonds, sesame seeds, tahini, figs, and oranges are a few plant foods that are relatively rich in calcium, with each serving containing up to 100 mg.

If plant-based diets are varied, and balanced, and comprise foods high in calcium and fortified goods, they can supply adequate levels of calcium. Nonetheless, certain people might still require calcium supplements, particularly if they have high calcium requirements, inadequate calcium absorption, or high calcium excretion. To meet their calcium needs, older folks, postmenopausal women, vegans, individuals with kidney illness, celiac disease, or inflammatory bowel disease, and athletes may find it helpful to take calcium supplements. Water-soluble vitamin B12 is necessary for the synthesis of red blood cells, DNA, and nerve cells. A lack of vitamin B12 can lead to anemia, brain damage, and cognitive decline. The recommended daily allowance (RDA) for vitamin B12 is 2.4 micrograms for adults and 2.8 micrograms for women who are pregnant or nursing.

Only animal items, including meat, eggs, and dairy, contain vitamin B12.,

Chapter 3: The Myth of Antioxidants

Free radicals are unstable chemicals that can cause oxidative damage to cells and tissues. Antioxidants are compounds that can stop or lessen this damage. Numerous meals, particularly fruits and vegetables, contain antioxidants, which may offer several health advantages. We must dispel several myths and misconceptions surrounding antioxidants. Here are a few of them:

Myth: All vitamins are antioxidants.

Fact: In addition to vitamins, additional substances with antioxidant qualities include minerals, enzymes, phytochemicals, and other substances. Antioxidants that are not vitamin-based include glutathione, lipoic acid, zinc, copper, manganese, selenium, flavonoids, carotenoids, and polyphenols. These antioxidants cooperate in various ways to shield the organism from the damaging effects of oxidative stress.

Myth: Antioxidants can prevent or cure diseases.

Factual statement: Antioxidants shield cells from oxidative damage and inflammation, which can help lower the chance of developing certain diseases like diabetes, cancer, cardiovascular disease, and neurological disorders. Antioxidants, however, are not panaceas that can treat or avoid illnesses on their own. They are a component of the intricate web of variables that affect health, which also includes nutrition, environment, lifestyle, and heredity. Furthermore, some research has indicated that using large amounts of antioxidant supplements may have negative consequences, including an increased risk of bleeding, cancer, and death.

Myth: An abundance of antioxidants is preferable.

Factual statement: Antioxidants are necessary to keep the body's defenses against free radicals and antioxidants in a healthy balance. On the other hand, having too little or too much of either might be harmful. Overconsumption of antioxidants can disrupt free radicals' ability to communicate, defend, and adapt as needed. Additionally, it may lessen the efficacy of certain drugs that use free radicals to kill cancer cells, like radiation and chemotherapy. Conversely, a low consumption of antioxidants can result in oxidative stress, which damages cells and tissues and speeds up the aging and illness processes. As a result, the ideal quantity of antioxidants varies depending on the requirements, health, and food intake of the individual.

Foods that are rich in antioxidants include the following:

Dark chocolate: The minerals and antioxidants in cocoa may reduce the risk of inflammation and heart disease.

Pecans: Rich in antioxidants, minerals, and healthy fats, they may lower cholesterol and increase blood antioxidant levels.

Blueberries are a low-calorie food that is high in minerals and antioxidants, particularly anthocyanins, which may shield the heart and brain from oxidative damage.

Strawberries: Rich in vitamin C and anthocyanins, which may help decrease blood pressure and LDL cholesterol, strawberries are sweet and adaptable fruits.

Artichokes are rich in antioxidants, minerals, and fiber, particularly chlorogenic acid, which may have anti-diabetic, anti-cancer, and anti-heart disease properties.

Goji berries: Due to their abundance of vitamins, minerals, and antioxidants like zeaxanthin, which may shield the eyes from age-related illnesses, goji berries are frequently promoted as a superfood.

These are but a few examples of foods rich in antioxidants. Antioxidants are also present in other fruits, vegetables, seeds, nuts, and legumes.

Consuming a diverse range of these items as part of a well-balanced diet may help you increase your antioxidant levels and fend off oxidative stress and chronic illnesses.

Part II: The Science of Brain Metabolism

The study of how the brain generates and uses energy to sustain its operations is known as brain metabolism science. Despite making up only 2% of the body mass, the brain is one of the most metabolically active organs in the body, using up 20% of all oxygen and glucose. The primary energy source for the brain is aerobic glycolysis, which breaks down glucose into pyruvate and acetyl-CoA, which enters the citric acid cycle and generates ATP, the cell's primary energy currency. Depending on availability and demand, the brain can also use additional substrates such as lactate, ketone bodies, and amino acids.

The electrical and chemical signaling of neurons and glia, which make up brain activity, is closely related to the metabolism of the brain. Synaptic transmission, or the transfer of neurotransmitters between neurons, is what drives brain activity. Energy is needed for synaptic transmission to produce and release neurotransmitters, recycle them, and maintain ion gradients across the membrane. The cerebral blood flow, which supplies oxygen and glucose to the brain tissue, is likewise influenced by brain activity. Numerous systems, including neurological, hormonal, and vascular ones, control the flow of blood in the brain.

The brain's metabolism is also regulated by several external and internal factors, such as nutrition, exercise, stress, age, and diseases. For instance, a diet heavy in fat and low in carbohydrates might cause ketosis, which is the body producing ketone bodies from fat. The brain can use ketone bodies as an alternate fuel, particularly when starving or fasting. Exercise can boost the expression of genes and proteins involved in energy metabolism and neuroprotection, as well as cerebral blood flow and oxygen transport. By triggering the hypothalamic-pituitary-adrenal axis, which releases chemicals like cortisol and adrenaline, stress can change the metabolism of the brain. These hormones have an impact on the brain's oxidative stress, inflammation, and absorption and utilization of glucose. By lowering antioxidant defense, blood-brain barrier integrity, and mitochondrial function, aging can affect brain metabolism. Disorders like stroke, Parkinson's disease, and Alzheimer's can impair brain metabolism by resulting in ischemia, inflammation, and neuronal degeneration. Understanding both normal and aberrant brain functioning, as well as creating novel approaches to the diagnosis, prevention, and therapy of brain illnesses, depends on the science of brain metabolism. Through a range of methods, including genetic engineering, biochemical analysis, brain imaging, and computer modeling, scientists can investigate the intricate relationships between brain activity and metabolism and how these are influenced by different circumstances. The study of brain metabolism can also highlight the potential benefits of metabolic therapies for improving brain function and health, including nutrition, exercise, medication, and gene therapy.

Chapter 4: The Role of Insulin Resistance in Brain Health

Insulin resistance is a disorder where the body's cells lose their sensitivity to the insulin hormone, which controls blood sugar levels. High blood glucose levels, which can harm the brain and other organs and tissues, are a result of insulin resistance. The brain's ability to operate can be hampered by insulin resistance, which also raises the risk of cognitive decline and neurodegenerative illnesses like Alzheimer's.

Numerous facets of brain health can be impacted by insulin resistance in the brain, including:

Metabolism: The process of using and creating energy to support brain activity is known as brain energy metabolism, and insulin plays a role in controlling it. The primary fuel for the brain, glucose, is absorbed and used by brain cells more easily when insulin is present. Insulin also affects how the brain uses other substrates, like lactate, amino acids, and ketone bodies, based on need and availability. The brain's insulin resistance can hinder the metabolism of glucose and other substrates, which can result in less energy being produced and more oxidative stress being experienced. Memory: The act of encoding, storing, and retrieving information is known as memory formation and consolidation, and insulin plays a part in this process. The ability of synapses, or the connections between neurons, to alter in strength and structure in response to experience and learning is known as synaptic plasticity, and insulin increases it. The expression of genes and proteins involved in the establishment and maintenance of memory is also modulated by insulin. Insulin resistance in the brain can affect memory performance and promote memory loss by compromising the molecular mechanisms of memory and synaptic plasticity.

Insulin signaling: Insulin binds to proteins on the surface of brain cells called insulin receptors, which then trigger intracellular signaling pathways. This is how insulin affects the brain. The hypothalamus, hippocampus, amygdala, and cortex are among the brain areas that express insulin receptors and are involved in the control of hunger, body weight, glucose homeostasis, emotion, and cognition. Reduced insulin action and altered insulin signaling can result from insulin resistance in the brain, which also lowers the quantity and functionality of insulin receptors. Research and clinical practice should focus on the role that insulin resistance plays in brain health because it may offer valuable information on the etiology and treatment of brain illnesses linked to metabolic dysfunction, including diabetes, obesity, and Alzheimer's disease. It may be possible to improve brain health and function by developing novel techniques for diagnosis, therapy, and intervention and by comprehending the causes and effects of insulin resistance in the brain.

Chapter 5:The Role of Ketones in Brain Health

Metabolites called ketones are created when the body uses fat as fuel, particularly in situations where glucose is in short supply. They can be utilized as a substitute for glucose, the brain's primary fuel source. Numerous impacts of ketones on brain function have been demonstrated, including control over gene expression, cell signaling, and neuronal excitability. According to some research, ketones may help treat neurological diseases like epilepsy, Alzheimer's, and brain damage.

Ketones and the Health of the Brain

The brain is an extremely intricate and energy-intensive organ that needs nourishment to function correctly continuously. Although glucose is the brain's principal fuel, the body can also use fat as an energy source when glucose is scarce, as occurs during fasting, exercise, or diabetes. Ketones are a byproduct of the breakdown of fat that is released into the bloodstream. The brain's cells can use ketones as an alternate fuel source since they can pass across the blood-brain barrier.

Ketones are active brain function modulators in addition to being passive energy carriers. They can impact several facets of neuronal physiology, including gene expression, cell signaling, and excitability. Ketones, for instance, can increase the activity of GABA, the primary inhibitory neurotransmitter in the brain, and decrease glutamate, the primary excitable neurotransmitter. Both a decrease in neuronal firing and a decrease in seizures may come from this. Additionally, transcription factors that control the expression of genes involved in neuroprotection, antioxidant defense, and synaptic plasticity can be activated by ketones. Ketones can also function as signaling molecules, regulating the activity of enzymes and receptors related to metabolism and neural communication.

Numerous neurological disorders that are typified by poor glucose metabolism, oxidative stress, inflammation, or neuronal damage may be affected by the impact of ketones on brain function. Ketones, for example, have been demonstrated to have anticonvulsant properties in cases of epilepsy, an illness characterized by aberrant brain activity that results in recurring convulsions. In Alzheimer's disease, a degenerative condition characterized by the buildup of amyloid plaques and neurofibrillary tangles in the brain that result in cognitive impairment and memory loss, ketones may also have neuroprotective effects. In cases of brain injury—a disorder that results in neuronal death and malfunction as a result of trauma, stroke, or hypoxia—ketone bodies may also have neurorestorative properties. Ketone supplementation—acquired by ingesting exogenous ketones or adhering to a ketogenic diet—is one method of raising the body's and the brain's amounts of ketones. A ketogenic diet is a high-fat, low-carb diet that stimulates the synthesis of ketones from fat and imitates the metabolic state of fasting. Since it was first introduced in the 1920s, ketones have been employed as a therapeutic approach for several neurological diseases, most notably epilepsy. More clinical trials are required to establish the ideal amount, duration, and manner of administration, and the effectiveness and safety of ketone supplementation for various neurological diseases are still being investigated.

Ketones are more than just a different kind of brain fuel. They have the power to significantly alter gene expression, cell signaling, and neuronal excitability in the brain. Ketones may be helpful for several neurological disorders linked to inflammation, oxidative stress, poor glucose metabolism, or neuronal damage. To fully understand the workings and potential effects of ketone supplementation on brain health, additional research is necessary.

Chapter 6: The Role of Essential Fatty Acids in Brain Health

The body needs to get essential fatty acids (EFAs) from food because it is unable to produce them. They consist of omega-3 (n-3) and omega-6 (n-6) polyunsaturated fatty acids (PUFAs). Because they are significant components of cell membranes, regulate the activity of several enzymes and receptors, and act as precursors for bioactive molecules, EFAs are involved in brain development, function, and aging.

EFAs and mental wellness

The brain is an extremely intricate and energy-intensive organ that needs a steady flow of fuel and nutrients to operate correctly. As they play a part in different aspects of neuronal physiology and disease, EFAs are among the nutrients that are crucial for brain health.

The two primary categories of EFAs are n-3 and n-6 PUFAs. Eicosapentaenoic acid (EPA) and docosahexaenoic acid (DHA) are the most significant n-3 PUFAs for the brain, whereas arachidonic acid (AA) is the most significant n-6 PUFA. These polyunsaturated fatty acids (PUFAs) originate from alpha-linolenic acid (ALA) and linoleic acid (LA), their respective predecessors, which are found in plant sources such as flaxseed, walnuts, soybean, and sunflower oils. Nevertheless, in humans, the conversion of ALA and LA to EPA, DHA, and AA is restricted and inefficient, and it is influenced by several variables, including age, gender, diet, and heredity. As a result, it is advised to eat meals high in EPA, DHA, and AA, such as meat, fish, seafood, and eggs, or to take supplements with fish oil or other PUFA sources.

Because they are absorbed into the phospholipids of cell membranes, particularly in the gray matter, where they affect the fluidity, permeability, and signaling properties of the membranes, EPA, DHA, and AA are crucial for brain development during both the prenatal and postnatal periods. Additionally, they have an impact on the expression and function of several proteins, including neurotrophins, growth factors, and synaptic proteins, which are involved in the development, differentiation, synaptogenesis, and plasticity of neurons. Furthermore, they serve as starting points for the manufacture of docosanoids, which include resolvins and neuroprotectins, and eicosanoids, which include prostaglandins, thromboxanes, and leukotrienes. These bioactive compounds control vascular function, inflammation, immunology, and neurotransmission in the brain.

Because they alter the action of several neurotransmitter systems, including dopamine, serotonin, glutamate, and GABA, which are involved in cognitive functions including learning, memory, attention, and mood, EPA, DHA, and AA are also crucial for brain function and aging. Additionally, they shield the brain against the damaging effects of oxidative stress, neuroinflammation, and neurodegeneration—disorders linked to aging and several neurological conditions, including depression, stroke, Parkinson's disease, and Alzheimer's disease. Higher intakes or levels of EPA, DHA, and AA have been linked in several studies to enhanced mental health, reduced risk of cognitive decline, and superior cognitive function in people. In summary, because they have a role in many facets of brain development, function, and aging, EFAs are critical for maintaining the health of the brain. Their levels and balance in the brain are influenced by several circumstances, and they can be supplied by diet or supplements. By affecting the synthesis and activity of different bioactive compounds, the expression and function of different proteins, and the structure and function of cell membranes, EFAs have positive effects on the brain.

Part III: The Power of Personalized Nutrition

The goal of the developing discipline of personalized nutrition research is to provide dietary recommendations that are specific to the individual's genetic makeup, microbiome, metabolic reactions, and lifestyle choices. The premise of personalized nutrition is that various individuals may react differently to the same foods or nutrients and that an individual's optimal diet may differ from that of another. Personalized nutrition offers more precise and focused dietary regimens to prevent or treat chronic diseases.

Personalized Nutrition's Power

One of the biggest things affecting our health and well-being is our nutrition. Nutrition, however, is not a science that is appropriate for all situations because various people have varied demands and dietary preferences. This is where customized nutrition enters the picture, providing a more exacting and tailored method to maximize our food consumption and health results. Personalized nutrition is a meal plan that is tailored to an individual's needs and goals based on a variety of data, including genetics, medical history, gut microbiota, metabolic responses, and lifestyle choices. For instance, based on an individual's genetic variants, blood levels, and metabolic reactions, customized nutrition can assist in determining the ideal macronutrients (proteins, fats, and carbs) and micronutrients (vitamins and minerals) in terms of amounts and types. A person's gut microbiota composition, food preferences, allergies, intolerances, and cultural background can all be taken into account when determining the optimal foods and dietary patterns through personalized nutrition.

By offering more efficient and focused dietary interventions, personalized nutrition holds the potential to enhance human well-being and prevent or treat several chronic illnesses, including diabetes, cancer, obesity, and cardiovascular disease. For example, by accounting for the fact that every individual reacts differently to the same meals, personalized nutrition can help balance blood sugar and blood fat levels, which are important risk factors for metabolic syndrome and cardiovascular disease. Because personalized nutrition considers the unique interactions that each person's gut microbiota has with various foods and nutrients, it can also help modify immunological function, oxidative stress, and inflammation—all of which are linked to several chronic diseases. By considering how various foods and nutrients affect each person's neurotransmitter systems, personalized nutrition can also aid in improving mental health, mood, and cognitive function.

The notion of personalized nutrition is dynamic and adaptive, subject to change over time due to the unique traits and demands of each individual based on a range of factors, including age, health state, environment, and lifestyle changes. Consequently, to gather, evaluate, and provide individualized nutrition recommendations, wearable technology, smartphone apps, artificial intelligence, and ongoing monitoring and feedback are all necessary for personalized nutrition. Research in the exciting and cutting-edge area of personalized nutrition has the potential to transform our food habits and enhance our overall health and well-being. Personalized nutrition can help us achieve optimal health and nutrition by providing more relevant and accurate dietary advice based on each individual's uniqueness and diversity.

Chapter 7: How to Evaluate Your Own Brain Health

The state of the brain that allows it to support many elements of cognition, including learning, memory, attention, and mood, is known as brain health. Numerous factors, including genetics, lifestyle, environment, and aging, might have an impact on brain health. Assessing your own mental well-being can assist you in determining your advantages and disadvantages, tracking your development, and implementing preventative or remedial measures to enhance your mental well-being.

How to Assess Your Own Mental Well-Being

It might be difficult to assess your own brain health because no one test or measurement can fully convey the diversity and complexity of the brain.

You can determine areas that require improvement and evaluate your current state of mental health with the aid of a few techniques and resources, though. Using online self-assessments, such as the Cogniciti Brain Health Assessment or the Cleveland Clinic Brain Check-up, is one way to test your memory and cognitive function. These evaluations can provide you with feedback and suggestions regarding the state of your brain because they are validated by experts and grounded in scientific research. Also, you can monitor your progress over time and contrast your outcomes with those of others. Nevertheless, if you have any worries or symptoms, you should still see a doctor because these evaluations are not meant to be diagnostic.

Keeping an eye on your lifestyle choices, such as how much sleep, food, exercise, stress, and social interaction you have, is another way to support brain health. You can track and evaluate your everyday actions and behaviors using a variety of methods, including wearable technology, smartphone apps, and journals. Additionally, you can track your accomplishments and development and create targets. You may determine what lifestyle behaviors are most effective for you and what needs to be modified or enhanced by monitoring your routines.

A third strategy is to expose your brain to novel and exciting activities that can improve your brain's plasticity and cognitive abilities. Some examples of these activities include taking a course, learning a new language, playing an instrument, or solving puzzles. To locate and access these activities, you can utilize a variety of resources, including books, websites, podcasts, and online courses. Additionally, you can gauge your progress and contentment by completing exams, questionnaires, or surveys. Your brain will remain robust and active if you provide it with challenges.

You can monitor your progress and changes, gain insight into your cognitive strengths and weaknesses, and take action to enhance your brain health by evaluating the health of your own brain. You may take control of the health and well-being of your brain by using online self-assessments, keeping an eye on your lifestyle choices, and mentally stimulating yourself.

Among the lifestyle choices that can enhance mental well-being are:

Maintaining social interactions with family, friends, and the community

Giving up tobacco use or limiting your exposure to smoke

Trying new and difficult things to keep your mind active, such as taking a course, playing a game, or learning a new skill,

Practicing stress management and relaxation methods like yoga, meditation, or breathing exercises
maintaining an active lifestyle, and engaging in moderate-to-intense exercise for a minimum of 150 minutes every week.
Maintaining a regular sleep schedule and getting enough sleep—aiming for at least seven hours—are important.
Consuming a diet low in added sugars, salt, and saturated fats and high in fruits, vegetables, whole grains, lean proteins, healthy fats, and water.
managing blood pressure, and blood sugar, and abstaining from excessive alcohol intake123
These practices can improve your mood, mental health, and cognitive function while shielding your brain from oxidative stress, inflammation, and neurodegeneration.

Among the meals that can improve the health and function of your brain are: Omega-3 fatty acids, which are abundant in oily fish like salmon, trout, tuna, herring, and sardines, help maintain and regenerate brain tissue, enhance mood and memory, and stave off cognitive decline.

Flavonoids, a class of antioxidants found in dark chocolate, have the ability to increase blood flow and neuron growth in the brain, boost mood, and improve cognitive abilities and adaptability.

Flavonoids found in berries, including blueberries, strawberries, raspberries, and blackberries, help lessen oxidative stress and inflammation in the brain, enhance learning and memory, and stave off age-related brain disorders.

Nuts and seeds that are rich in vitamin E, a powerful antioxidant that can shield the brain from oxidative damage, as well as minerals, proteins, and healthy fats that can promote brain function, including walnuts, almonds, sunflower, and pumpkin seeds.

Whole grains, like quinoa, barley, brown rice, and oats, are excellent providers of B vitamins, fiber, and complex carbs that can help the body produce neurotransmitters, control blood sugar, and give the brain consistent energy.

Caffeine and antioxidants included in coffee can improve mood, alertness, focus, and cognitive function while reducing the risk of Parkinson's and Alzheimer's disease.

Avocados contain vitamin K, folate, and vitamin C, which can prevent blood clots and improve cognitive function. They are also high in monounsaturated fats, which can increase blood flow and lower blood pressure in the brain.

Peanuts include resveratrol, a polyphenol that can shield the brain from oxidative stress and inflammation, and they're also high in niacin, a B vitamin that can prevent cognitive decline and boost memory.

Eggs contain lutein and zeaxanthin, two carotenoids that can enhance visual and cognitive performance, and they are rich in protein and choline, a nutrient that can boost the synthesis of acetylcholine, a neurotransmitter that is crucial for memory and communication among brain cells.

Broccoli includes glucosinolates, which are substances that can alter the activity of several enzymes and receptors in the brain, in addition to being high in vitamin K, a fat-soluble vitamin that can improve memory and cognitive function.

In addition to iron, calcium, and magnesium that help support brain development, kale is rich in vitamins A, C, and K that can shield the brain from oxidative stress, inflammation, and neurodegeneration.

Soy includes lecithin, a phospholipid that can enhance the integrity and fluidity of brain cell membranes and is high in protein. Phytoestrogens are plant substances that can mimic the effects of estrogen, a hormone that can affect mood, memory, and cognition.

These are a few foods that can improve the condition and functionality of your brain. But it's crucial to keep in mind that sustaining optimal brain health also requires a varied and balanced diet in addition to other lifestyle aspects like exercise, sleep, and stress reduction.

Among the meals that may harm the structure and functionality of your brain are:

Sugar-filled beverages, like fruit juice, sports drinks, energy drinks, and soda, can lower brain capacity, induce inflammation in the brain, raise the risk of dementia, and affect memory and learning.

refined carbs, which can raise blood sugar levels, cause inflammation, and affect cognitive function; examples of these are white bread, pasta, rice, and pastries.

Trans fats can lower brain volume, raise the risk of Alzheimer's disease, and impair memory. They are present in some margarine, baked products, fast food, and processed foods.

processed foods: rich in nitrates, preservatives, and salt, processed meats like bacon, ham, salami, and sausages can harm the brain, impair cognition, and raise the risk of stroke.

Alcohol can alter neurotransmitters, decrease the brain, deteriorate memory, and raise the chance of dementia.

Fish high in mercury, like king mackerel, swordfish, shark, and tuna, can build up in the brain and cause Alzheimer's disease, neurological damage, and cognitive impairment.

These are a few foods that may be detrimental to the health and function of your brain. It's crucial to keep in mind that balance and moderation are essential and that occasionally consuming certain meals might not have a major negative impact on your mental well-being.

Chapter 8: How to Choose the Best Diet for Your Brain

Selecting the optimal diet for your brain can be difficult because there are a lot of things to take into account, including your age, goals, tastes, and health. Making wise decisions that are good for your brain can be aided by a few broad rules and recommendations.

How to Pick the Healthiest Diet for Your Mind

The most intricate and important organ in your body, your brain, needs an ongoing flow of nourishment and energy to function correctly. Your brain's functionality and health, as well as your chance of contracting certain neurological conditions like Alzheimer's, Parkinson's, and stroke, can be greatly influenced by the foods you eat. Consequently, selecting the optimal food for your brain is crucial for both your general health and cognitive function. However, since every individual may have unique genetic, metabolic, and environmental elements that affect their brain health, no one diet can meet everyone's needs and preferences. Based on the most recent research findings and professional advice, there are a few broad concepts and suggestions that might assist you in selecting the optimal diet for your brain. Among them are:

Consuming a wide range of foods high in vitamins, minerals, phytochemicals, omega-3 fatty acids, antioxidants, and other nutrients can shield your brain from oxidative stress, inflammation, and neurodegeneration. Fatty fish, berries, nuts, seeds, dark chocolate, green leafy vegetables, coffee, and tea are some of the healthiest meals for your brain. Avoiding or reducing the number of foods heavy in alcohol, trans fats, refined carbs, added sugars, and salt, as these foods can harm the brain, raise the risk of dementia, and impair memory. The worst foods for your brain are processed meats, sugar-filled beverages, white bread, pastries, and mercury-filled seafood. Adhering to a nutritious, balanced, diverse, and moderate dietary pattern that emphasizes plant-based foods, whole foods, and healthy fats while minimizing animal products, processed foods, and saturated fats. The DASH diet, MIND diet, Nordic diet, and Mediterranean diet are a few dietary regimens that have been linked to improved brain function. Customizing your diet to your unique needs, including age, health, preferences, and objectives; speaking with your physician or a nutritionist about any particular ailments or worries that might have an impact on the health of your brain. Additionally, you can assess your brain health and receive individualized suggestions by using online tools like the Cleveland Clinic Brain Check-up and the Cogniciti Brain Health Assessment.

Selecting the ideal diet for your brain can help you avoid or postpone the beginning of several neurological disorders, as well as improve your mood, mental health, and cognitive function. It can be a difficult but worthwhile procedure. You may make wise decisions for your brain and get the rewards of tasty and nutritious food by adhering to these concepts and recommendations.

What is the diet known as the Mediterranean diet?

The traditional foods of Mediterranean countries like Greece, Italy, France, and Spain form the basis of the Mediterranean diet, which is a healthy eating pattern. It places a focus on fruits, vegetables, whole grains, legumes, nuts, seeds, olive oil, fish, and shellfish, in addition to dairy, eggs, poultry, and wine in moderation. It also restricts processed meals, salt, added sugars, and red meat. Heart disease, diabetes, and Alzheimer's are just a few of the chronic diseases that the Mediterranean diet may help prevent or treat.

The following are a few advantages of the Mediterranean diet:

It can improve your mood, mental health, and cognitive performance while shielding your brain from oxidative stress, inflammation, and neurodegeneration.

By enhancing blood lipid profile, blood sugar levels, and blood vessel function, it can reduce the risk of cardiovascular disease, stroke, and high blood pressure.

By offering you nutrient-dense, satisfying foods and lowering your consumption of calories, fat, and sugar, it can assist you in controlling your weight and preventing obesity.

Chapter 9: How to Optimize Your Diet for Your Brain

Since nutrition and energy are essential for the healthy operation of the brain, the health and performance of your brain can be greatly influenced by the foods you eat. You must take into account several aspects, including your age, health state, preferences, goals, and the type, quantity, and quality of the foods you eat, to optimize your diet for your brain.

How to Eat to Boost Your Brain Function

The brain is the body's most intricate and important organ, and it needs a steady flow of nourishment and energy to function correctly. Your diet has an impact on the health and function of your brain as well as your chance of contracting certain neurological conditions like stroke, Parkinson's disease, and Alzheimer's.

As a result, eating a diet that is optimized for your brain is crucial for both your general health and cognitive function. However, since every individual may have unique genetic, metabolic, and environmental elements that affect their brain health, no one diet can meet everyone's needs and preferences. Nonetheless, based on the most recent research findings and professional advice, there are a few broad concepts and recommendations that might assist you in optimizing your diet for your brain. Among them are:

Eating a range of foods high in vitamins, minerals, phytochemicals, omega-3 fatty acids, antioxidants, and other nutrients can improve your mental, emotional, and cognitive health, as well as shield your brain from oxidative stress, inflammation, and neurodegeneration. Fatty fish, berries, nuts, seeds, dark chocolate, green leafy vegetables, coffee, and tea are some of the healthiest meals for your brain.

restricting or avoiding diets heavy in alcohol, trans fats, processed carbs, added sugars, and salt, as these can raise the risk of dementia, deteriorate memory, and damage the brain. The worst foods for your brain are processed meats, sugar-filled beverages, white bread, pastries, and mercury-filled seafood. Adhering to a nutritious, balanced, diverse, and moderate dietary pattern that emphasizes plant-based foods, whole foods, and healthy fats while minimizing animal products, processed foods, and saturated fats. The DASH diet, MIND diet, Nordic diet, and Mediterranean diet are a few dietary regimens that have been linked to improved brain function.

customizing your diet to your unique needs, including age, health, tastes, and aspirations; speaking with a doctor or nutritionist about any particular issues or ailments that might have an impact on the health of your brain. Additionally, you can assess your brain health and receive individualized suggestions by using online tools like the Cleveland Clinic Brain Check-up and the Cogniciti Brain Health Assessment. A brain-friendly diet can help you avoid or postpone the beginning of several neurological disorders, as well as enhance your mood, mental health, and cognitive function. You may make wise decisions for your brain and get the rewards of tasty and nutritious food by adhering to these concepts and recommendations. Supplements marketed as enhancing or protecting brain function, memory, mood, or focus are known as brain-boosting supplements. They may have negative effects or interfere with other medications, and the evidence for their safety and efficacy is frequently insufficient or nonexistent. As a result, you should always get medical advice before taking any supplements, particularly if you have any health issues. Among the most typical components of supplements that enhance cognitive **function are:**

Fish, nuts, seeds, and other plant oils contain omega-3 fatty acids, which are important lipids. They may protect against cognitive decline, improve blood flow, and lower inflammation to promote the health of your brain. The advantages of omega-3 supplements are unclear, though, and not everyone may benefit from them.

B vitamins: The body uses these water-soluble vitamins for several metabolic functions, including the synthesis of neurotransmitters and the upkeep of nerve cells. Certain brain illnesses, including depression and Alzheimer's disease, may be prevented or treated with their assistance. Supplementing with B vitamins can have variable effects, though, depending on your nutritional state and genetic makeup.

One stimulant that can improve your alertness, focus, mood, and cognitive function is caffeine. Coffee, tea, chocolate, and certain energy beverages and supplements all include it. Caffeine, however, can also have negative consequences, including headaches, insomnia, and anxiety. Moreover, individuals with high blood pressure, heart issues, or sleep disorders might not want to use caffeine.

Ginkgo biloba: Traditional Chinese medicine has been using this herb for generations. It might guard against oxidative stress and neurodegeneration and enhance blood flow and oxygen supply to the brain. Additionally, it might improve cognitive and memory abilities, particularly in older people. Supplementing with ginkgo, however, has conflicting data and can have negative effects like bleeding, allergic reactions, and drug interactions.

Another herb that has been utilized for generations in traditional Asian medicine is ginseng. It may enhance mood, memory, and mental function in addition to having neuroprotective, antioxidant, and anti-inflammatory properties. However, there is a huge range in the quality and amount of ginseng supplements, and they may mix with other drugs and cause adverse effects like headaches, sleeplessness, and gastrointestinal issues.

There are numerous supplements that can improve cognitive function; some of the most well-known ones are creatine, curcumin, resveratrol, and bacopa monnieri. All of these supplements might not be effective for everyone, and none of them is a panacea for brain health. Maintaining a healthy lifestyle, which includes eating a balanced diet, getting regular exercise, getting enough sleep, managing stress, and engaging in social and mental activities, is the best approach to maintaining the health of your brain.

Conclusion

How to Feed, Guard, and Recharge Your Brain.

This book has taught you how nutrition affects brain function and how to design a diet that is best for your brain. You now know the truth about some of the myths and misconceptions surrounding brain food, including the use of antioxidants, superfoods, supplements, and plant-based diets. You have also studied the science of brain metabolism and the effects of various nutrients on brain health and function, including insulin, ketones, and essential fatty acids. Ultimately, you now understand the significance of customized nutrition and how to assess, select, and tailor your diet to your unique needs, objectives, and features.

You may make wise decisions for your brain and get the rewards of tasty and nutritious food by adhering to the concepts and recommendations in this book. It is also possible to enhance your mood, mental health, and cognitive performance, as well as postpone or prevent the start of several neurological conditions, including Parkinson's, Alzheimer's, and stroke. You can also reach your full mental capacity and improve your performance, creativity, and productivity.

Recall that your brain requires the finest nutrition and care since it is the most intricate and important organ in your body. You may enhance not only the health and function of your brain but also your general well-being and quality of life by making dietary changes that are best for your brain.